CW00515533

Keto Diet Cookbook 2021

-Easy and Delicious Ketogenic Diet Recipes -

[Dr. Dean Chasey]

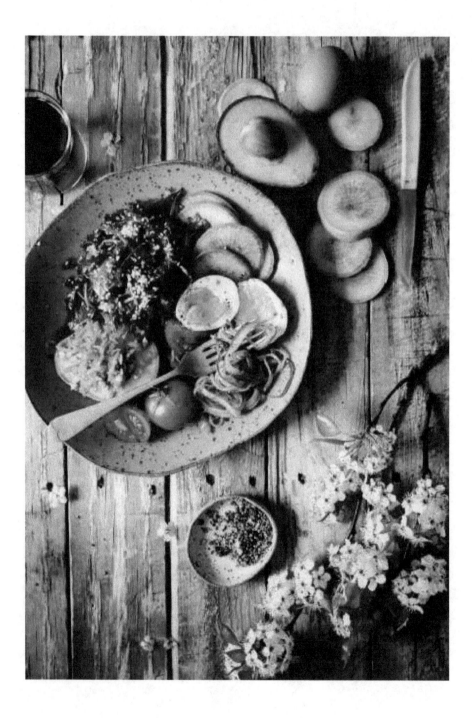

Table Of Content

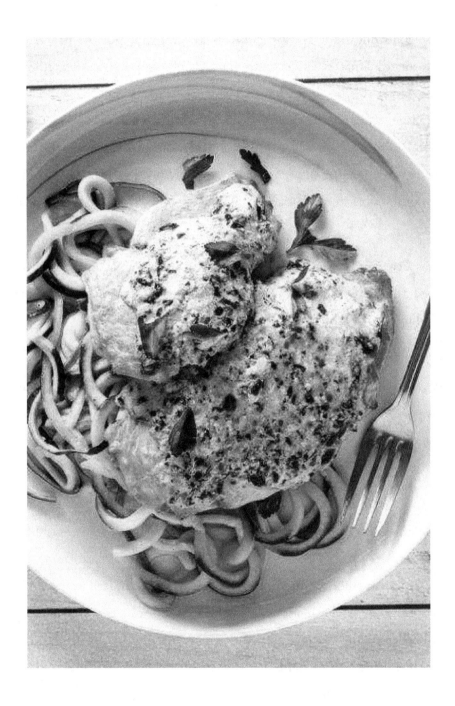

Additionally, the information in the following pages is intended only for informational purposes and should thus be thought of as universal. As befitting its nature, it is presented without assurance regarding its prolonged validity or interim quality. Trademarks that are mentioned are done without written consent and can in no way be considered an endorsement from the trademark holder.

CHAPTER 1: **BREAKFAST**

Lemon Crepes

0:40 Prep
0:20 Cook
Makes 8

INGREDIENTS

1 cup (150g) plain flour, sifted
White sugar, to serve
Pinch of salt
1 1/4 cups (310ml) milk
15g butter, melted
2 eggs
Lemon wedges, to serve

METHOD

1

Place sifted plain flour and a pinch of salt in a large mixing bowl. Make
a well in the centre.

2

In a separate bowl, use a balloon whisk to mix together the eggs, milk
and melted butter.

3

Pour the milk mixture into flour and whisk, gradually incorporating
the flour until smooth and well combined. Cover and refrigerate for 30
minutes.

4

Heat an 18-20cm crepe pan or small frying pan over a medium heat.
Lightly grease with butter. Pour 1/4 cup (60ml) crepe batter into the
pan and swirl to coat the base. Cook for 2 minutes or until golden and
lacy. Turn over and cook for a further 30 seconds. Transfer to a plate

and repeat with the remaining batter. Serve scattered with white sugar and a lemon wedge.

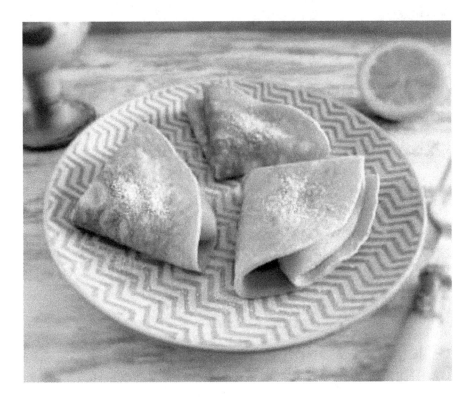

Seeded Morning Loaf

Servings:

24

Yield:

2 - 9x5 inch loaves

Ingredients

3 cups all-purpose flour

2 cups white sugar

¾ teaspoon salt

¾ cup butter, softened

3 eggs

½ cup lemon juice

¾ cup plain yogurt

½ cup poppy seeds

3 tablespoons lemon zest

1 ½ teaspoons baking soda

Directions

1

Preheat oven to 350 degrees F. Heavily grease and flour two 9x5 inch loaf pans.

2

Sift together flour, baking soda, and salt. Set aside.

3

In a large bowl, cream butter or margarine, and sugar until light and fluffy. Beat in eggs, one at a time.

4

Mix lemon juice and yogurt together and add alternately with the sifted flour mixture to the butter mixture. Mix until just blended. Stir in lemon rind and poppy seeds. Pour mixture into prepared pans and smooth tops.

5

Bake at 350 degrees F for 50-55 minutes or until browned and a knife inserted in the center comes out clean. Cool on rack for 15 minutes before turning out of pans.

Nutrition

Per Serving: 203 calories; protein 3.4g; carbohydrates 30.4g; fat 7.9g; cholesterol 39mg; sodium 207.3mg.

Canadian Eggs Benedict

Prep:

25 mins

Cook:

5 mins

Total:

30 mins

Servings:

4

Yield:

4 servings

Ingredients

4 egg yolks

8 strips Canadian-style bacon

3 ½ tablespoons lemon juice

1 pinch ground white pepper

2 tablespoons butter, softened

1 tablespoon water

1 cup butter, melted

¼ teaspoon salt

8 eggs

⅛ teaspoon Worcestershire sauce

1 teaspoon distilled white vinegar

4 English muffins, split

Directions

1

To Make Hollandaise: Fill the bottom of a double boiler part-way with water. Make sure that water does not touch the top pan. Bring water to a gentle simmer. In the top of the double boiler, whisk together egg yolks, lemon juice, white pepper, Worcestershire sauce, and 1 tablespoon water.

2

Add the melted butter to egg yolk mixture 1 or 2 tablespoons at a time while whisking yolks constantly. If hollandaise begins to get too thick, add a teaspoon or two of hot water. Continue whisking until all butter is incorporated. Whisk in salt, then remove from heat. Place a lid on pan to keep sauce warm.

3

Preheat oven on broiler setting. To Poach Eggs: Fill a large saucepan with 3 inches of water. Bring water to a gentle simmer, then add vinegar. Carefully break eggs into simmering water, and allow to cook for 2 to 3 minutes. Yolks should still be soft in center. Remove eggs from water with a slotted spoon and set on a warm plate

4

While eggs are poaching, brown the bacon in a medium skillet over medium-high heat and toast the English muffins on a baking sheet under the broiler.

5

Spread toasted muffins with softened butter, and top each one with a slice of bacon, followed by one poached egg. Place 2 muffins on each plate and drizzle with hollandaise sauce. Sprinkle with chopped chives and serve immediately.

Nutrition

Per Serving: 879 calories; protein 31.8g; carbohydrates 29.6g; fat 71.1g; cholesterol 742.1mg; sodium 1719.3mg.

Lettuce Wrap Tacos

Prep:

20 mins

Cook:

22 mins

Total:

42 mins

Servings:

4

Yield:

4 servings

Ingredients

1 small onion, chopped

1 clove garlic, chopped

1 tablespoon taco seasoning mix

2 tablespoons olive oil

¾ cup chicken broth

salt and ground black pepper to taste

1 (16 ounce) garbanzo beans, drained and rinsed

1 avocado, sliced

1 tomato, chopped

1 (3 ounce) can sliced black olives

1 head iceberg lettuce, halved

½ teaspoon ground cumin

Directions

1

Heat olive oil in a large skillet. Add onion; cook and stir until translucent, about 4 - 6 minutes. Add garlic; cook and stir until fragrant, about 2 minutes.

2

Stir garbanzo beans, taco seasoning, and cumin into the skillet. Pour in chicken broth and cover. Bring to a boil; reduce heat to low and simmer until soft, about 10 minutes. Mash mixture with potato masher. Season with salt and pepper.

3

Pull lettuce "cups" out of the center of each half. Fill with garbanzo bean mixture. Top with avocado, tomato, and olives.

Nutrition

Per Serving: 344 calories; protein 8.8g; carbohydrates 40.2g; fat 18.1g; cholesterol 0.9mg; sodium 927.4mg.

Creamy Kale Omelet

Prep:

30 mins

Total:

30 mins

Servings:

2

Yield:

2 servings

Ingredients

2 slices OSCAR MAYER Bacon, chopped

½ pound kale, stems removed, leaves cut into 1/2-inch wide strips

1 tablespoon milk

2 teaspoons butter

½ cup KRAFT Shredded Triple Cheddar Cheese with a TOUCH OF PHILADELPHIA

¼ teaspoon ground black pepper

1 teaspoon GREY POUPON Dijon Mustard

4 eggs

Directions

1

Cook and stir bacon in small nonstick skillet until crisp. Remove bacon from skillet with slotted spoon, reserving 1 tsp. drippings in skillet. Drain bacon on paper towels. Add kale to reserved drippings; cook on medium heat 5 to 6 min. or just until kale is wilted. Transfer to bowl; wipe skillet clean.

2

Whisk eggs, milk and mustard until blended. Melt butter in same skillet on medium heat. Add egg mixture; cook 5 to 7 min. or until almost set, occasionally lifting edge with spatula to allow uncooked portion to flow underneath. Top with cheese; cook until egg mixture is set but top is still slightly moist.

3

Spoon kale onto half the omelet; top with bacon and pepper. Slip spatula underneath omelet, tip skillet to loosen and gently fold omelet in half. Slide or flip omelet onto plate; cut in half.

Nutrition

Per Serving: 386 calories; protein 21.8g; carbohydrates 13.6g; fat 28.6g; cholesterol 358.1mg; sodium 560.6mg.

Cream Cheese and Tomato Omelet with Chives

Prep:

10 mins

Cook:

10 mins

Total:

20 mins

Servings:

1

Yield:

1 omelet

Ingredients

2 eggs
2 tablespoons seeded and diced tomato
1 tablespoon milk
3 tablespoons cream cheese, softened
1 tablespoon chopped fresh chives
salt and ground black pepper to taste

Directions

1

Whisk eggs, milk, salt, and pepper together in a bowl.

2

Heat a 6-inch nonstick skillet over medium heat; pour egg mixture into the hot skillet, tilting so egg mixture covers the entire bottom of skillet. Slowly cook egg mixture until set, 5 to 10 minutes.

3

Arrange small dollops of cream cheese onto half the omelet; sprinkle tomato and chives over cream cheese. Fold omelet in half over the fillings. Remove skillet from heat and cover until cream cheese has softened, 2 to 3 minutes.

Nutrition

Per Serving: 260 calories; protein 15.6g; carbohydrates 3.1g; fat 20.8g; cholesterol 406.2mg; sodium 236.1mg.

Baked Omelet

Prep:

15 mins

Cook:

40 mins

Total:

55 mins

Servings:

4

Yield:

4 servings

Ingredients

8 eggs

1 tablespoon dried minced onion

1 cup milk

½ cup shredded Cheddar cheese

½ teaspoon seasoning salt

3 ounces cooked ham, diced

½ cup shredded mozzarella cheese

Directions

1

Preheat oven to 350 degrees F. Grease one 8x8 inch casserole dish and set aside.

2

Beat together the eggs and milk. Add seasoning salt, ham, Cheddar cheese, Mozzarella cheese and minced onion. Pour into prepared casserole dish.

3

Bake uncovered at 350 degrees F for 40 to 45 minutes.

Nutrition

Per Serving: 314 calories; protein 24.8g; carbohydrates 5.9g; fat 21.2g; cholesterol 415.3mg; sodium 738.2mg.

Fruit Kefir Smoothie

Prep:

5 mins

Total:

5 mins

Servings:

1

Yield:

1 smoothie

Ingredients

½ cup kefir

½ small banana

1 tablespoon almond butter

½ cup frozen blueberries

2 teaspoons honey

Directions

1

Combine kefir, blueberries, banana, almond butter, and honey in a blender. Process until smooth.

Nutrition

Per Serving: 306 calories; protein 7.2g; carbohydrates 42.3g; fat 14.2g; sodium 127.5mg.

Croque Madame with Poached Eggs

Prep:

10 mins

Cook:

10 mins

Total:

20 mins

Servings:

2

Yield:

2 sandwiches

Ingredients

6 slices avocado

4 slices Dietz & Watson Maple Honey Ham

2 eggs

1 tablespoon white vinegar

3 slices Dietz & Watson Swiss Cheese

1 English muffin

Directions

1

Cut the top off the English muffin, using the muffin as the base for the Croque Madame.

2

Place three slices of avocado on each muffin base, then place the Dietz & Watson Swiss Cheese on top. Place the Dietz & Watson Maple Honey Ham on top of that.

3

Prepare a pot for the eggs. Fill a shallow saucepan with three inches of water and bring it to a simmer.

4

Crack 1 egg into the saucepan and add distilled white vinegar to the water. Turn down the heat until the bubbles disappear. Use a wooden spoon to make the water swirl, keeping egg at the center of the whirlpool. Cook for 3 minutes and remove with a slotted spoon. The yolk should wiggle, but shouldn't be too loose. Repeat with the second egg.

5

Place eggs over the ham. Poke eggs a little bit to allow the yolk to run down each muffin.

Nutrition

Per Serving: 508 calories; protein 32.5g; carbohydrates 23.9g; fat 27.3g; cholesterol 254mg; sodium 708.8mg.

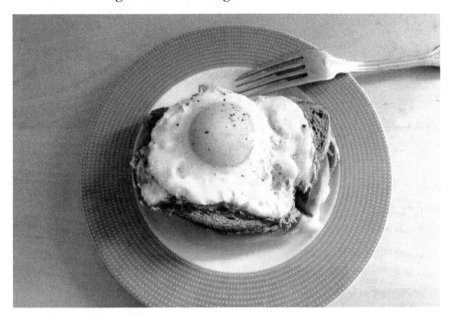

Keto Vanilla Milkshake

Prep:

5 mins

Total:

5 mins

Servings:

1

Yield:

1 serving

Ingredients

1 scoop vanilla ice cream

⅛ teaspoon vanilla extract

1 cup half-and-half cream

Directions

1

In a blender, combine ice cream, half-and-half and vanilla extract. Blend until smooth. Pour into glass and serve.

Nutrition

Per Serving: 358 calories; protein 7.9g; carbohydrates 15.4g; fat 30.1g; cholesterol 98.8mg; sodium 116.1mg.

Caprese Omelet

Prep:

25 mins

Total:

25 mins

Servings:

2

Yield:

2 servings

Ingredients

2 plum tomatoes, thickly sliced

1 tablespoon balsamic vinegar

1 avocado, cubed

½ cup green olives

½ cup canned artichoke hearts, drained and chopped

2 tablespoons torn fresh basil leaves

salt and ground black pepper to taste

½ English cucumber, peeled and sliced

3 (4 ounce) balls buffalo mozzarella, thickly sliced

2 tablespoons olive oil

Directions

1

Divide tomatoes, mozzarella, avocado, cucumber, green olives, artichoke hearts, and basil between two serving plates, layering them in that order. Season with salt and pepper.

2

Drizzle olive oil and balsamic vinegar over layers.

Nutrition

Per Serving: 631 calories; protein 44.1g; carbohydrates 13.3g; fat 45.2g; cholesterol 108.9mg; sodium 2150.4mg.

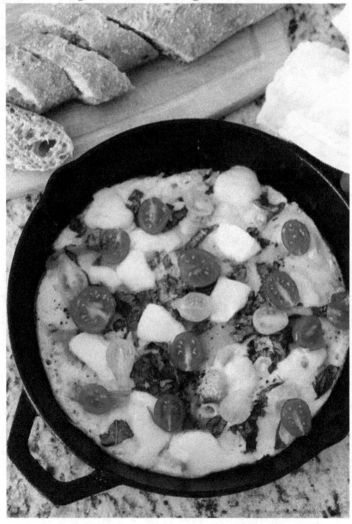

CHAPTER 2: SOUPS & SALAD

Buffalo Chicken Soup

Prep:

15 mins

Cook:

20 mins

Total:

35 mins

Servings:

8

Yield:

8 servings

Ingredients

¼ cup butter

1 small onion, diced

¼ cup all-purpose flour

¾ cup half-and-half cream

3 cups water

¼ cup buffalo wing sauce

1 cube chicken bouillon

2 cups cubed cooked chicken

1 ½ cups shredded Cheddar cheese

3 stalks celery, diced

salt and pepper to taste

Directions

1

Melt the butter in a large pot over medium-high heat; cook the celery and onion in the melted butter until tender, about 5 minutes. Add the flour and allow to cook until absorbed, about 2 minutes more. Slowly stir the half-and-half and water into the mixture. Dissolve the bouillon in the liquid. Stir in the chicken, buffalo wing sauce, and Cheddar cheese. Season with salt and pepper. Reduce heat to medium-low. Stirring occasionally, allow the soup to simmer until the the cheese has melted completely, about 10-12 minutes.

Nutrition

Per Serving: 259 calories; protein 16.5g; carbohydrates 6.9g; fat 18.3g; cholesterol 72.2mg; sodium 570mg.

Artichoke Salad

Prep:

15 mins

Cook:

20 mins

Total:

35 mins

Servings:

4

Yield:

4 servings

Ingredients

1 (10.75 ounce) package chicken flavored rice mix (e.g. Rice A Roni)

½ cup mayonnaise

1 tablespoon Worcestershire sauce

2 (6.5 ounce) jars marinated artichoke hearts, diced

1 tablespoon lemon juice

6 green onions, chopped

12 pimento-stuffed green olives, chopped

1 green bell pepper, chopped

1 teaspoon curry powder

1 dash hot pepper sauce

Directions

1

Prepare rice as package directs, omitting butter, instead spray pan with non-stick vegetable oil. Cool mixture in refrigerator.

2

In a mixing bowl, combine artichokes, green onions, green olives and bell pepper.

3

Prepare the dressing by whisking together the mayonnaise, Worcestershire sauce, lemon juice, curry powder and hot pepper sauce. Pour dressing over combined rice and vegetable mix, stir well and chill.

Nutrition

Per Serving: 608 calories; protein 8.4g; carbohydrates 63.8g; fat 38.6g; cholesterol 10.4mg; sodium 1872.1mg.

Kale Soup

Servings:

12

Yield:

12 servings

Ingredients

1 medium onion, chopped

1 pound Portuguese chourico, broken into large chunks

3 cloves garlic, minced

4 tablespoons olive oil

2 (15 ounce) cans kidney beans, drained

1 (15 ounce) can garbanzo beans, drained

2 pork chops

salt and pepper

3 tablespoons Pimenta Moida (Portuguese hot chopped peppers)

1 bunch kale - washed, dried, and shredded

5 Yukon Gold potatoes, cubed

½ head savoy cabbage, shredded

Directions

1

In a large soup pot, cook onion and garlic in olive oil over medium heat until soft. Mix in choirico, beans, and potatoes, and then add pork chops to the pot. Season with salt and pepper, and add enough water to the pan to cover all of the **Ingredients**. Bring to a boil, then reduce heat, and simmer until potatoes are tender.

2

Once potatoes are tender, taste soup, add Pimenta Moida and more salt and pepper. Stir in kale and cabbage, and increase heat to gently boil. Kale only needs about 5 minutes. You may add some water if the soup got too thick, I like this soup on the brothy side.

Nutrition

Per Serving: 348 calories; protein 17.3g; carbohydrates 33g; fat 17.1g; cholesterol 36.4mg; sodium 617.7mg.

CHAPTER 3: LUNCH

Peanut Butter, Mayonnaise, and Lettuce Sandwich

Prep:

5 mins

Total:

5 mins

Servings:

1

Yield:

1 sandwich

Ingredients

2 slices bread

2 tablespoons peanut butter

2 lettuce leaves

1 tablespoon mayonnaise

Directions

1

Spread one slice of bread with mayonnaise. Spread the other slice with peanut butter. Place lettuce leaves on top of the peanut butter, then top with the mayonnaise-side of the other piece of bread to make a sandwich.

Nutritions

Per Serving: 428 calories; protein 12.4g; carbohydrates 33g; fat 29g; cholesterol 5.2mg; sodium 571.2mg.

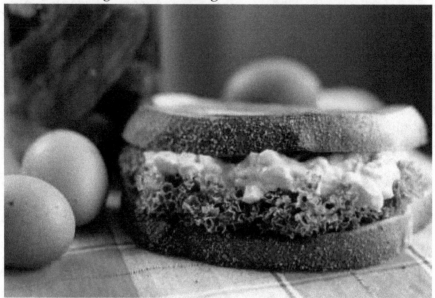

Chicken Inasal

Prep:

30 mins

Cook:

38 mins

Total:

1 hr 8 mins

Servings:

4

Yield:

4 servings

Ingredients

2 teaspoons garam masala

2 teaspoons tandoori masala powder

2 teaspoons Madras curry powder

½ teaspoon ground cardamom

½ teaspoon ground cayenne pepper

salt and ground black pepper to taste

1 ½ pounds boneless, skinless chicken thighs, cut into bite-size pieces

3 tablespoons butter, divided

1 teaspoon ground cumin

1 yellow onion, chopped

4 cloves garlic, minced

2 teaspoons chopped fresh ginger

1 cup tomato puree

1 cup half-and-half

1 tablespoon lemon juice

¼ cup plain yogurt

⅓ cup cashews
1 bunch fresh cilantro, stems removed

Directions

1

Mix garam masala, tandoori masala, curry, cumin, cardamom, cayenne, salt, and black pepper together in a small bowl to make spice mixture.

2

Place chicken in a large bowl and add 1/2 the spice mixture; turn to coat evenly.

3

Melt 1 tablespoon butter in a large skillet over medium heat. Add chicken; cook and stir until lightly browned, about 10 minutes. Remove from heat.

4

Melt remaining 2 tablespoons butter in a large saucepan over medium heat. Add onion; cook and stir until soft and translucent, about 5 minutes. Stir in remainder of the spice mixture, lemon juice, garlic, and ginger; cook and stir until combined, about 1 minute.

5

Stir tomato puree into onion mixture and cook, stirring frequently, about 2 minutes. Pour in half-and-half and yogurt. Reduce heat to low and simmer sauce, stirring frequently, about 10 minutes. Remove from heat.

6

Blend cashews in a blender until finely ground. Add sauce to the blender; puree until smooth.

7

Pour blended sauce over chicken in the skillet. Simmer until thickened, 10 to 15 minutes. Garnish with cilantro.

Nutritions

Per Serving: 552 calories; protein 33.2g; carbohydrates 22g; fat 38g; cholesterol 142mg; sodium 541.7mg.

Country Captain Chicken

Prep:

25 mins

Cook:

1 hr 50 mins

Total:

2 hrs 15 mins

Servings:

8

Yield:

8 servings

Ingredients

1 whole whole chicken, cut into 8 pieces

3 tablespoons Madras curry powder

1 teaspoon ground thyme

kosher salt and freshly ground black pepper to taste

¼ cup canola oil

6 slices applewood smoked bacon, chopped

1 large yellow onion, diced small

2 cups cooked basmati rice

3 ribs celery, chopped

4 cloves garlic, minced

1 (28 ounce) can whole peeled tomatoes, drained and chopped, liquid reserved

¼ cup dried currants, plus more for garnish

2 green bell peppers, chopped

¼ cup golden raisins

2 tablespoons unsalted butter

2 bay leaves

2 tablespoons peanuts

2 tablespoons chopped fresh parsley

Directions

1

Season chicken with thyme, kosher salt, and black pepper.

2

Heat oil in a 5-quart Dutch oven over high heat. Place chicken pieces, skin-side down, in hot oil and cook until golden brown, 2 to 5 minutes. Transfer chicken to a plate; drain and discard oil.

3

Reduce heat to medium and add bacon to the Dutch oven. Cook and stir until bacon is browned and crispy, 8 to 10 minutes. Transfer bacon to a paper towel-lined plate. Chop into smaller pieces.

4

Cook and stir onion, celery, bell peppers, and garlic in the Dutch oven over medium heat until soft, about 10 minutes. Add chopped tomatoes, 3/4 cup reserved tomato liquid, currants, raisins, curry powder, butter, bay leaves, salt, and black pepper; bring to a simmer, reduce heat to medium-low, cover the Dutch oven with a lid, and simmer until sauce is thickened, about 30 minutes.

5

Preheat oven to 325 degrees F.

6

Return chicken to Dutch oven and spoon sauce over the top. Cover the Dutch oven with a lid.

7

Bake in the preheated oven until chicken is tender, about 1 hour. An instant-read thermometer inserted into the thickest part of the thigh, near the bone should read 165 degrees F.

8

Press 1/2 cup rice into a small bowl and invert onto a plate to remove. Set 2 pieces of chicken on rice and spoon sauce over the top. Repeat with remaining rice, chicken, and sauce. Garnish each with bacon, currants, peanuts, and parsley.

Nutritions

Per Serving: 783 calories; protein 28.2g; carbohydrates 28.9g; fat 62g; cholesterol 105.7mg; sodium 471.1mg.

Grilled Spiced Chicken

Ingredients

1 teaspoon ground ginger

2 tablespoons dark rum

½ teaspoon ground cinnamon

¼ teaspoon ground cumin

1 dash cayenne pepper

4 skinless, boneless chicken breast halves

2 cups water

1 cup basmati rice

1 mango - peeled, seeded and diced

¼ teaspoon ground anise seed

½ cup orange juice

2 tablespoons honey

2 teaspoons cornstarch

1 ½ tablespoons water

2 tablespoons fresh lime juice

Directions

1

In a medium bowl, mix the ginger, cinnamon, cumin, anise, and cayenne pepper. Rub the chicken with the spice mixture, and place in the bowl. Cover, and refrigerate 20 to 30 minutes.

2

Combine 2 cups of water and basmati rice in a saucepan, and bring to a boil. Reduce heat, cover and simmer for 20 minutes, or until tender.

3

In a small saucepan, mix the mango, orange juice, lime juice, and honey. Bring to a boil, reduce heat, and simmer for 5 minutes, stirring occasionally. In a small cup, mix cornstarch with 1 1/2 tablespoons of water until cornstarch is dissolved. Stir into mango mixture, and simmer one minute, or until sauce has thickened slightly. Stir in dark rum.

4

Preheat an outdoor grill for medium heat. When grill is hot, brush the grate with oil.

5

Grill chicken 6 to 8 minutes per side, until no longer pink and juices run clear. Serve over the cooked rice, and top with the mango sauce.

Nutritions

Per Serving: 418 calories; protein 28.9g; carbohydrates 62.4g; fat 3.5g; cholesterol 67.2mg; sodium 66.2mg.

Thai Pork Meal

Prep:

5 mins

Cook:

20 mins

Total:

25 mins

Servings:

5

Yield:

5 servings

Ingredients

1 tablespoon vegetable oil

2 ½ cups Thai-style coconut curry stir-fry sauce (such as KanTong®)

1 ¼ pounds lean pork, cut into cubes

Directions

1

Heat oil in a large saucepan over high heat; cook pork in hot oil until completely browned, about 5 minutes.

2

Pour stir-fry sauce into the saucepan, bring to a simmer, and cook until the pork is cooked through, 15 to 20 minutes.

Nutritions

Per Serving: 224 calories; protein 23g; carbohydrates 3.3g; fat 12.6g; cholesterol 63.2mg; sodium 435.6mg.

Beef Mini Meatloaves

Prep:

15 mins

Cook:

45 mins

Total:

1 hr

Servings:

8

Yield:

8 servings

Ingredients

1 egg

¼ cup packed brown sugar

¾ cup milk

½ cup quick cooking oats

1 teaspoon salt

1 pound ground beef

1 cup shredded Cheddar cheese

⅔ cup ketchup

1 ½ teaspoons prepared mustard

Directions

1

Preheat oven to 350 degrees F.

2

In a large bowl, combine the egg, milk, cheese, oats and salt. Add the ground beef, mixing well, and form this mixture into eight miniature meatloaves. Place these in a lightly greased 9x13 inch baking dish.

3

In a separate small bowl, combine the ketchup, brown sugar and mustard. Stir thoroughly and spread over each meatloaf.

4

Bake, uncovered, at 350 degrees F for 45 minutes.

Nutritions

Per Serving: 255 calories; protein 15.1g; carbohydrates 16.6g; fat 14.4g; cholesterol 73.9mg; sodium 656mg.

Pan-Fried Chive Flowers

Prep:

10 mins

Cook:

5 mins

Total:

15 mins

Servings:

2

Yield:

2 servings

Ingredients

1 tablespoon olive oil

1 ½ cups fresh chive flowers, rinsed and well-drained

1 clove garlic, minced

salt

black pepper

1 tablespoon butter

Directions

1

Heat olive oil in a large skillet over medium-high heat. Add butter; heat until melted, about 30 seconds. Add chive flowers, garlic, and salt; cook and stir until soft and tender, 3 to 5 minutes. Grind black pepper over mixture before serving.

Nutritions

Per Serving: 125 calories; protein 1.4g; carbohydrates 2.4g; fat 12.8g; cholesterol 15.3mg; sodium 120.1mg.

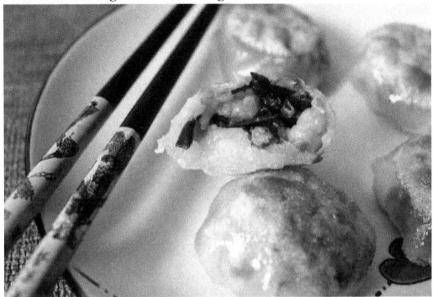

Halibut Steaks with Corn and Chanterelles

Prep:

20 mins

Cook:

20 mins

Total:

40 mins

Servings:

2

Yield:

2 servings

Ingredients

2 large halibut steaks

salt and ground black pepper to taste

2 tablespoons olive oil

1 cup corn kernels

⅓ cup diced roasted red peppers

½ cup water

2 cups sliced chanterelle mushrooms

1 tablespoon butter

1 tablespoon minced fresh tarragon

1 lemon, juiced

Directions

1

Preheat grill for medium-high heat and lightly oil the grate. Season halibut steaks with salt and black pepper.

2

Heat olive oil in a skillet over medium heat. Cook and stir chanterelle mushrooms with a pinch of salt in hot oil until soft and caramelized, about 10 minutes. Stir corn and peppers into mushrooms until corn is toasted, about 2 minutes.

3

Pour water into mushroom mixture; bring to a simmer and cook until reduced, about 5 minutes. Stir lemon juice and butter into mushroom mixture until butter melts and liquid is almost evaporated.

4

Cook halibut steaks on the preheated grill until until the fish flakes easily with a fork, 3 to 5 minutes per side. Divide mushroom mixture between two plates and sprinkle tarragon over each. Top mushrooms with halibut steaks.

Nutritions

Per Serving: 562 calories; protein 53.6g; carbohydrates 30.9g; fat 25.7g; cholesterol 86.8mg; sodium 339.1mg.

Super Short Ribs

Prep:

30 mins

Cook:

2 hrs

Total:

2 hrs 30 mins

Servings:

8

Yield:

8 servings

Ingredients

1 tablespoon olive oil

2 onions, quartered

1 (8 ounce) can pineapple chunks

1 (14 ounce) can beef broth

½ cup chili sauce

4 ¼ pounds beef short ribs

¼ cup honey

4 cloves garlic, minced

salt and pepper to taste

2 tablespoons chopped fresh parsley, for garnish

3 tablespoons Worcestershire sauce

Directions

1

Preheat oven to 350 degrees F.

2

Heat the oil in a Dutch oven over medium high heat. Add the ribs and brown well on all sides in small batches. Set ribs aside.

3

Add the onions, broth, pineapple, chili sauce, honey, Worcestershire sauce and garlic. Return the ribs to the pot, coating them well with this sauce.

4

Bake, covered, at 350 degrees F for 1 hour. Remove cover, season with salt and pepper to taste, and bake for 1 more hour. Garnish with the parsley.

Nutritions

Per Serving: 600 calories; protein 24.3g; carbohydrates 21.7g; fat 46.1g; cholesterol 99.1mg; sodium 507.7mg.

Smoked Salmon and Lettuce Bites

Prep:

20 mins

Total:

20 mins

Servings:

6

Yield:

6 servings

Ingredients

2 cups mayonnaise

1 (3 ounce) package smoked salmon, flaked

½ lemon, juiced

2 tablespoons chopped capers

2 Granny Smith apples, cored and sliced

1 ½ cups sweet corn

3 tablespoons chopped fresh dill

Directions

1

Mix mayonnaise, lemon juice, dill, and capers together in a large bowl until smooth. Add apples, corn, and smoked salmon; toss gently until evenly coated. Chill before serving.

Nutritions

Per Serving: 603 calories; protein 4.9g; carbohydrates 17.8g; fat 59.2g; cholesterol 31.1mg; sodium 615.7mg.

CHAPTER 4: DINNER

North African Paella

Prep:

35 mins

Cook:

18 mins

Additional:

10 mins

Total:

1 hr 3 mins

Servings:

6

Yield:

6 servings

Ingredients

¼ cup olive oil

1 onion, chopped

1 roasted red pepper, chopped

2 cloves garlic, chopped

3 vine-ripened tomatoes, chopped

1 (8 ounce) salmon fillet, cut into pieces

5 ounces merguez sausage, cut into pieces

6 cups vegetable broth, divided

½ cup white wine

1 teaspoon ground cumin

salt and ground black pepper to taste

12 shrimp, shelled and deveined

12 mussels, cleaned and debearded

2 (5.8 ounce) boxes couscous

Directions

1

Heat olive oil in a large pot over medium heat. Add onion, roasted red pepper, and garlic; cook and stir until fragrant, 3 to 4 minutes. Stir in tomatoes, salmon fillet, and merguez sausage; cook for 2 to 3 minutes.

2

Pour 2 1/2 cups broth and white wine into the pot. Season stew with cumin, salt, and pepper; bring to a boil. Reduce heat to low and stir in shrimp; simmer until opaque, about 3 minutes. Remove from heat and add mussels; cover and let stand until mussels open, about 5 minutes.

3

Bring remaining 3 1/2 cups broth to a boil in a separate pot. Stir in couscous. Remove from heat and let stand until couscous absorbs broth, about 5 minutes.

4

Serve couscous in shallow bowls; ladle stew on top.

Nutrition

Per Serving: 519 calories; protein 30.3g; carbohydrates 55.8g; fat 16.8g; cholesterol 76.4mg; sodium 707.3mg.

Red Wine Chicken

Prep:

10 mins

Cook:

30 mins

Additional:

1 hr

Total:

1 hr 40 mins

Servings:

2

Yield:

2 servings

Ingredients

1 cup red wine
½ cup balsamic vinaigrette salad dressing
2 skinless, boneless chicken breast halves
salt and pepper to taste
3 shallots, finely chopped
½ teaspoon chopped fresh thyme leaves

Directions

1

Pour the red wine and vinaigrette into a resealable plastic bag. Sprinkle the chicken breasts with salt and pepper, and place into the bag. Coat the chicken with the marinade, squeeze out excess air, and seal the bag. Marinate in the refrigerator for at least 1 hour.

2

Pour the marinade into a skillet over high-medium heat, and cook, stirring frequently, until the marinade begins to reduce and the oil separates, about 15 minutes. Place the chicken into the skillet and brown on both sides, about 4 minutes per side. Stir in the shallots, and cook, stirring, until translucent, about 10 minutes. Stir in the thyme leaves and cook until the sauce is reduced and the chicken is browned and no longer pink in the center, about 4 to 5 minutes.

Nutrition

Per Serving: 459 calories; protein 25.5g; carbohydrates 21.7g; fat 20.8g; cholesterol 64.6mg; sodium 769.9mg.

Caribbean Beef

Prep:

10 mins

Cook:

6 mins

Additional:

2 hrs 30 mins

Total:

2 hrs 46 mins

Servings:

6

Yield:

6 steaks

Ingredients

1 fluid ounce coconut-flavored rum

¼ teaspoon salt

¼ teaspoon ground black pepper

⅛ teaspoon ground cinnamon

½ teaspoon garlic powder

½ teaspoon dried oregano

¼ teaspoon dried sage

½ teaspoon white vinegar

1 tablespoon fresh lemon juice

4 slices onion

6 (8 ounce) beef top sirloin steaks

1 tablespoon olive oil

Directions

1

Whisk together the rum, salt, pepper, cinnamon, powder, oregano, sage, vinegar, and lemon juice in a bowl; pour into a gallon-sized, resealable plastic bag. Add the onion and steaks to the marinade. Seal the bag, squeezing out as much air as possible. Allow to marinate in refrigerator 2 1/2 hours.

2

Heat the olive oil in a large skillet over medium heat. Cook the steaks with the skillet covered to desired doneness, about 3 minutes per side for medium rare.

Nutrition

Per Serving: 381 calories; protein 37.3g; carbohydrates 2.3g; fat 23.1g; cholesterol 122.4mg; sodium 183.9mg.

Beef Empanadas

Prep:

15 mins

Cook:

35 mins

Total:

50 mins

Servings:

10

Yield:

10 servings

Ingredients

1 tablespoon vegetable oil

1 pound ground beef or turkey

1 medium onion, chopped

½ teaspoon salt

1 (10.75 ounce) can Campbell's® Condensed Black Bean, Cumin & Cilantro Soup

4 ounces queso fresco, crumbled

1 (14 ounce) package empanada dough, thawed

1 egg, beaten

Directions

1

Heat the oven to 425 degrees F.

2

Heat the oil in a 12-inch skillet over medium-high heat. Add the beef, onion and salt and cook until the beef is well browned, stirring often to separate meat. Pour off any fat.

3

Reduce the heat to medium. Stir the soup in the skillet and cook until the mixture is hot and bubbling. Remove the skillet from the heat. Stir in the queso fresco.

4

Spoon about 1/3 cup beef mixture in the center of each dough circle. Brush the edges of the dough circles with water. Fold the dough in half over the filling. Crimp the edges with a fork to seal. Brush the empanadas with the egg. Place the empanadas onto a baking sheet.

5

Bake for 20 minutes or until the empanadas are golden brown.

Nutrition

Per Serving: 290 calories; protein 13.9g; carbohydrates 25.8g; fat 14.7g; cholesterol 56.3mg; sodium 568.6mg.

South-American Shrimp

Prep:

10 mins

Cook:

20 mins

Total:

30 mins

Servings:

3

Yield:

3 servings

Ingredients

1 (12 fluid ounce) can evaporated milk

½ cup yellow grits

½ cup chicken broth

1 tablespoon salted butter

⅓ cup grated sharp Cheddar cheese

3 slices bacon

¾ cup frozen bell peppers

⅓ pound frozen medium shrimp - thawed, shelled, and deveined

½ teaspoon taco seasoning mix

2 teaspoons hot sauce, or to taste (Optional)

Directions

1

Combine evaporated milk, grits, chicken broth, and butter in a saucepan over medium-high heat; bring to a boil. Cook, stirring constantly, until thickened, 5 to 7 minutes. Add Cheddar cheese and stir until incorporated. Remove from the heat and set aside.

2

Place bacon in a large skillet and cook over medium-high heat, turning occasionally, until crisp and browned, about 3 minutes per side. Drain bacon slices on paper towels and chop when cool enough to handle.

3

Add bell peppers to the bacon grease. Add shrimp and taco seasoning. Cook and stir until peppers are heated through and shrimp are bright pink on the outside and the meat is opaque, 3 to 5 minutes. Stir in chopped bacon.

4

Place a dollop of grits in each bowl and top with shrimp mixture and hot sauce.

Nutrition

Per Serving: 469 calories; protein 27.2g; carbohydrates 39.7g; fat 22.3g; cholesterol 147.5mg; sodium 866.7mg.

Zoodle Bolognese

Prep:

20 mins

Cook:

2 hrs 40 mins

Total:

3 hrs

Servings:

8

Yield:

8 servings

Ingredients

4 ounces pancetta bacon, finely diced

3 carrots, finely diced

3 stalks celery, finely diced

2 onions, finely diced

3 tablespoons extra-virgin olive oil

1 pound 85% lean ground beef

1 pound ground pork

½ cup dry white wine

1 (28 ounce) can San Marzano whole peeled tomatoes, drained

½ teaspoon ground nutmeg

½ teaspoon salt

¼ teaspoon crushed red pepper

1 cup beef stock

¼ cup heavy cream

1 (16 ounce) box tagliatelle pasta

¼ cup grated Parmesan cheese, or to taste

Directions

1

Cook pancetta in a pan over medium heat until it has released its fat and is crisp, 7 to 8 minutes. Add carrots, celery, and onions and cook until the vegetables soften and the onions are translucent, 7 to 8 minutes. Set aside.

2

Heat olive oil in a 4-quart pot over medium heat. Break ground beef and pork into small chunks and add them to the pot; cook, stirring lightly, until browned, 7 to 8 minutes.

3

Stir the pancetta-vegetable mixture into the ground meat. Add wine. Reduce heat to medium-low and stir, breaking up the meat until finely ground, wine has evaporated, and the pot is almost dry, 13 to 15 minutes. Add tomatoes, nutmeg, salt, and red pepper. Use the back of a spoon to break up the tomatoes and continue to break down the meat mixture into very small bits, about 5 minutes.

4

Pour beef stock and heavy cream into the pot and reduce heat to the lowest setting. Leave to simmer, partially covered, stirring occasionally, for at least 2 hours.

5

Meanwhile, fill a large pot with lightly salted water and bring to a rolling boil. Cook tagliatelle at a boil until tender yet firm to the bite, about 8 minutes. Reserve 1 cup of pasta water and drain well.

6

Stir pasta into the Bolognese sauce and mix well, adding a little reserved pasta water if needed to develop a satiny coating. Top with grated Parmesan cheese.

Nutrition

Per Serving: 607 calories; protein 34.3g; carbohydrates 54.9g; fat 26.9g; cholesterol 94.6mg; sodium 543.9mg.

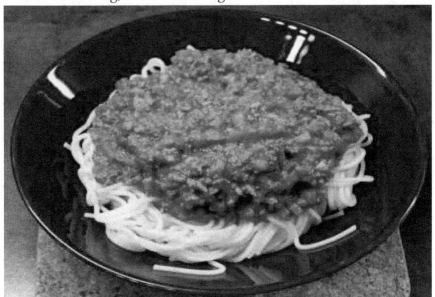

Fennel Cucumber Salsa

Prep:

20 mins

Additional:

20 mins

Total:

40 mins

Servings:

16

Yield:

4 cups

Ingredients

1 English cucumber, diced

2 tablespoons honey

1 large fennel bulb, diced

½ red onion, chopped

½ cup pickled banana peppers, diced

salt and pepper to tastE

1 bunch cilantro, chopped

1 avocado - peeled, pitted, and diced

3 tablespoons fresh lemon juice

Directions

1

Combine the cucumber, fennel, avocado, red onion, banana peppers, cilantro, honey, lemon juice, salt, and pepper in a bowl. Allow mixture to sit 20 minutes before serving.

Nutrition

Per Serving: 43 calories; protein 0.9g; carbohydrates 6.8g; fat 2g; sodium 18.4mg.

Wine Shrimp Scampi Pizza

Prep:

20 mins

Cook:

25 mins

Total:

45 mins

Servings:

3

Yield:

3 servings

Ingredients

12 ounces angel hair pasta

½ teaspoon cayenne pepper

¼ cup olive oil

2 tablespoons butter

½ yellow onion, diced

4 cloves garlic, minced

2 tablespoons chopped fresh cilantro

1 small tomato, diced

¼ cup olives, chopped

¼ cup chopped leeks

½ lemon, juiced

2 teaspoons capers

2 teaspoons salt

¼ cup Chardonnay wine

1 pound uncooked medium shrimp, peeled and deveined

¼ cup heavy whipping cream

Directions

1

Bring a large pot of lightly salted water to a boil. Cook angel hair pasta in the boiling water, stirring occasionally, until tender yet firm to the bite, 4 to 5 minutes. Drain.

2

Heat olive oil and butter in a large skillet over medium heat. Add onion and garlic; cook until onion is transparent, about 4 minutes. Add tomato, olives, Chardonnay wine, leeks, lemon juice, capers, salt, and cayenne pepper. Bring to a boil. Mix in shrimp and simmer until pink, about 10 minutes. Stir in heavy whipping cream and cilantro. Serve on top of angel hair pasta.

Nutrition

Per Serving: 796 calories; protein 38.5g; carbohydrates 72.5g; fat 38.8g; cholesterol 277.6mg; sodium 2272.1mg.

Shirataki Noodles

Prep:

10 mins

Cook:

25 mins

Total:

35 mins

Servings:

3

Yield:

3 servings

Ingredients

2 (8 ounce) packages shirataki noodles, drained and rinsed

1 tablespoon olive oil

2 cloves garlic, minced

¼ teaspoon red pepper flakes

12 ounces raw shrimp, peeled and deveined

¼ teaspoon salt

⅛ teaspoon ground black pepper

1 tablespoon minced shallot

3 tablespoons fresh lemon juice

2 tablespoons butter

1 tablespoon chopped fresh parsley

3 tablespoons dry white wine

Directions

1

Cover shirataki noodles with water and bring to a boil. Boil for 5 minutes. Drain.

2

Return drained noodles to the saucepan and cook over medium heat to remove any excess moisture, 5 to 6 minutes. Remove from heat and set aside.

3

Drizzle olive oil into a large skillet over medium heat. Add shallot and stir until translucent, 2 to 3 minutes. Take care not to burn. Add garlic and red pepper flakes; stir for 1 minute. Add shrimp and cook for 2 to 3 minutes per side, taking care not to overcook. Season with salt and pepper.

4

Transfer shrimp to a bowl, reserving pan drippings in the skillet. Whisk lemon juice and white wine into the skillet. Add butter and cook until fully incorporated and sauce begins to thicken slightly, 3 to 4 minutes.

5

Return shrimp to the skillet. Add noodles. Sprinkle with parsley and toss to combine.

Nutrition

Per Serving: 224 calories; protein 19g; carbohydrates 6.8g; fat 13.2g; cholesterol 190.7mg; sodium 461.4mg.

CHAPTER 5: Appetizer, Snacks & Side Dishes

Jalapeno Salsa

Prep:

15 mins

Cook:

12 mins

Total:

27 mins

Servings:

25

Yield:

3 cups

Ingredients

10 fresh jalapeno peppers
2 tomatoes
1 white onion, quartered
¼ cup chopped fresh cilantro, or more to taste
2 cloves garlic, smashed
1 lime, juiced
1 teaspoon salt
1 teaspoon ground black pepper

Directions

1

Place jalapenos in a saucepan with enough water to cover. Bring to a boil. Simmer until jalapenos soften and begin to lose their shine, about 10 to 12 minutes. Remove the jalapenos with a slotted spoon, chop off the stem, and place them in a blender. Add the tomatoes and boil for 2 to 3 minutes to loosen the skin. Peel the skin from the tomatoes and add tomatoes to the blender.

2

Place the onion, cilantro, garlic, lime juice, salt, and black pepper in the blender with the jalapenos and tomatoes. Blend to desired consistency.

Nutrition

Per Serving: 7 calories; protein 0.3g; carbohydrates 1.6g; fat 0.1g; sodium 94.1mg.

Wrapped Halloumi in Bacon

Prep:

10 mins

Cook:

15 mins

Total:

25 mins

Servings:

24

Yield:

24 breadsticks

Ingredients

2 (11 ounce) containers refrigerated breadstick dough

24 strips thinly-sliced bacon

1 cup grated Parmesan cheese

2 teaspoons garlic powder

Directions

1

Preheat oven to 375 degrees F (190 degrees C). Line 2 baking sheets with parchment paper.

2

Separate refrigerated dough into individual breadsticks. Wrap a strip of bacon around each one, tucking bacon ends underneath. Arrange on prepared baking sheets.

3

Bake in the preheated oven until golden brown, 15 to 20 minutes.

4

Mix Parmesan cheese and garlic powder together in a shallow dish. Roll breadsticks in the mixture while they are still warm.

Nutrition

Per Serving: 139 calories; protein 6.8g; carbohydrates 13.1g; fat 6.2g; cholesterol 13.2mg; sodium 459.9mg.

Sweet and Spicy Dipping Sauce

Prep:

5 mins

Cook:

15 mins

Additional:

15 mins

Total:

35 mins

Servings:

16

Yield:

1 cup

Ingredients

½ cup rice wine vinegar
½ cup white sugar
2 teaspoons salt
1 tablespoon chili garlic sauce (such as Lee Kum Kee®)

Directions

1

Stir the vinegar and sugar together in a small saucepan over medium heat until the sugar dissolves completely, 7 to 10 minutes; add the salt, reduce heat to low, and simmer until the mixture thickens slightly, about 5 minutes. Remove from heat and stir the chili garlic sauce into the mixture. Allow to cool slightly before serving.

Nutrition

Per Serving: 25 calories; carbohydrates 6.3g; sodium 330.4mg.

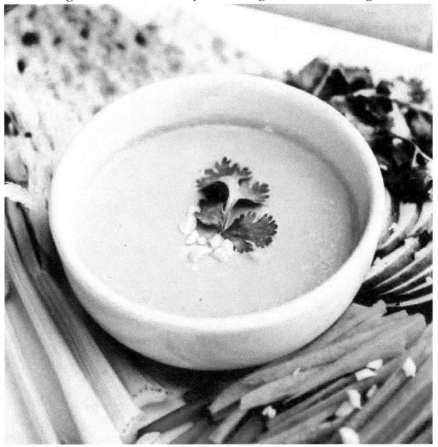

CHAPTER 6: Vegan & Vegetarian

Tempeh Taco Cups

Prep:

15 mins

Cook:

15 mins

Total:

30 mins

Servings:

4

Yield:

4 servings

Ingredients

2 tablespoons extra virgin olive oil

2 tablespoons taco seasoning mix

1 small onion, minced

1 (8 ounce) package spicy flavored tempeh, coarsely grated

½ cup vegetable broth

1 teaspoon dried oregano

2 cloves garlic, minced

Directions

1

Heat oil in skillet on medium-high heat. Cook and stir onion in the hot oil until it begins to soften, about 5 minutes; add garlic and continue to cook until fragrant, 1 to 2 minutes. Stir grated tempeh into onion mixture; cook and stir until lightly browned, about 5 minutes.

2

Pour vegetable broth over the tempeh mixture and reduce heat to low; season with taco seasoning, oregano, and ground red pepper. Cook, stirring regularly, until most of the liquid has evaporated, about 5 minutes.

Nutrition

Per Serving: 199 calories; protein 10.9g; carbohydrates 11.4g; fat 13g; sodium 391.6mg.

Cranberry Parfait

Prep:

20 mins

Additional:

3 hrs 15 mins

Total:

3 hrs 35 mins

Servings:

10

Yield:

10 servings

Ingredients

1 (14.5 ounce) can whole berry cranberry sauce
½ (14.4 ounce) package graham crackers
½ teaspoon vanilla extract
8 ounces heavy whipping cream
2 teaspoons white sugar
1 (14 ounce) can jellied cranberry sauce

Directions

1

Chill a large metal bowl in the refrigerator or freezer, about 17 minutes.

2

Mix whole berry cranberry sauce and jellied cranberry sauce together in a bowl.

3

Place graham crackers in a large resealable plastic bag and crush with a rolling pin into crumbs.

4

Pour heavy cream into the chilled bowl and whip with an electric mixer on high speed until soft peaks form, about 2 minutes. Add sugar and vanilla extract; whip until medium peaks form, about 2 minutes more.

5

Place half of the graham cracker crumbs in the bottom of a trifle bowl. Top with half of the cranberry mixture and whipped cream. Repeat layers, ending with whipped cream. Chill until set, at least 3 hours.

Nutrition

Per Serving: 287 calories; protein 2g; carbohydrates 47.7g; fat 10.5g; cholesterol 31.1mg; sodium 152.3mg.

Beanie-Weenie

Prep:

15 mins

Cook:

30 mins

Total:

45 mins

Servings:

6

Yield:

6 servings

Ingredients

1 (16 ounce) package hot dogs , cut into 1/4-inch slices

⅔ cup ketchup

1 ½ teaspoons garlic powder

1 (28 ounce) can baked beans with pork

1 tablespoon chopped fresh parsley

2 tablespoons cider vinegar

¼ cup Worcestershire sauce

Directions

1

In a large skillet, combine the hot dogs, baked beans, ketchup, cider vinegar, Worcestershire sauce, garlic powder and parsley. Mix to blend, and bring to a boil. Turn heat to low, cover, and simmer for 25 to 30 minutes, stirring occasionally.

Nutrition

Per Serving: 433 calories; protein 16g; carbohydrates 40.5g; fat 24.1g; cholesterol 48.9mg; sodium 1702.8mg.

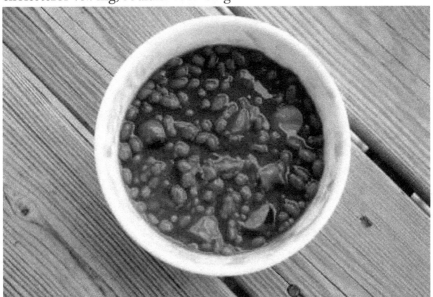

Spinach Egg White Muffins

Prep:

10 mins

Cook:

20 mins

Total:

30 mins

Servings:

10

Yield:

10 mini muffins

Ingredients

cooking spray

2 (4 ounce) cartons liquid egg whites

1 (10 ounce) package frozen chopped spinach, thawed and drained

1 teaspoon hot sauce

1 teaspoon salt

6 ounces shredded reduced-fat sharp Cheddar cheese

½ teaspoon ground black pepper

Directions

1

Preheat the oven to 350 degrees F. Spray a muffin tin with cooking spray.

2

Mix egg whites, Cheddar cheese, spinach, hot sauce, salt, and pepper in a bowl. Ladle mixture into the muffin tin, filling each cup 3/4 the way full.

3

Bake in the preheated oven until a knife inserted in the center of a muffin comes out clean, 20 to 25 minutes. Serve warm or cooled.

Nutrition

Per Serving: 59 calories; protein 8.2g; carbohydrates 1.8g; fat 2.2g; cholesterol 3.8mg; sodium 405.1mg.

CHAPTER 7: Desserts

Coffee Cake

Prep:

25 mins

Cook:

40 mins

Additional:

30 mins

Total:

1 hr 35 mins

Servings:

8

Yield:

1 9x12-inch cake

Ingredients

Dry **Ingredients**:

2 cups all-purpose flour

½ teaspoon fine sea salt

1 teaspoon baking powder

2 teaspoons unsalted butter

¾ teaspoon baking soda

Crumble Mixture:

1 ½ cups finely chopped toasted walnuts

⅓ cup white sugar

¼ teaspoon salt

⅓ cup packed light brown sugar

1 teaspoon ground cinnamon

3 tablespoons unsalted butter, melted

Wet **Ingredients**:

½ cup unsalted butter, at room temperature

2 large eggs

1 cup plain yogurt

1 cup white sugar

2 each Honeycrisp apples

1 ½ teaspoons vanilla extract

Directions

1

Preheat oven to 350 degrees F. Butter a 9x12-inch baking dish generously.

2

Whisk flour, sea salt, baking powder, and baking soda together in a bowl. Set aside.

3

Combine walnuts, brown sugar, white sugar, salt, cinnamon, and melted butter in a bowl. Mix until walnuts and sugar are thoroughly coated with butter.

4

Cream butter and sugar together in another bowl with a spatula until well blended. Add 1 egg and whisk until mixture is smooth, 2 to 3 minutes. Whisk in second egg until thoroughly incorporated. Add vanilla extract and yogurt; whisk together. Add flour mixture to wet **Ingredients**; whisk just until flour disappears. Do not overmix.

5

Remove cores from apples. Cut across into 1/8- to 1/4-inch slices. Stack up a few slices, make 1 cut down the center, and dice across into cubes. Add to cake batter, folding in with a spatula until just combined.

6

Spread 1/2 of the batter evenly into the bottom of the prepared baking dish. Scatter 1/2 of the crumble mixture evenly over the top. Top with the rest of the batter in dollops. Spread carefully to evenly distribute, trying not to disturb the crumbs. Top with the rest of the crumb mixture. Press crumbs into the batter very gently.

7

Bake in the center of the preheated oven until a toothpick or bamboo skewer inserted into the center comes out clean, about 40 minutes. Let cool to room temperature, about 30 minutes, before slicing and serving.

Nutrition

Per Serving: 631 calories; protein 9.6g; carbohydrates 76g; fat 34.1g; cholesterol 95mg; sodium 434.9mg.

Chocolate Ganache

Prep:

10 mins

Cook:

10 mins

Total:

20 mins

Servings:

16

Yield:

2 cups

Ingredients

1 cup heavy cream
9 ounces bittersweet chocolate, chopped

Directions

1

Place the chocolate into a medium bowl. Heat the cream in a small sauce pan over medium heat. Bring just to a boil, watching very carefully because if it boils for a few seconds, it will boil out of the pot. When the cream has come to a boil, pour over the chopped chocolate, and whisk until smooth. Stir in the rum if desired.

2

Allow the ganache to cool slightly before pouring over a cake. Start at the center of the cake and work outward. For a fluffy frosting or chocolate filling, allow it to cool until thick, then whip with a whisk until light and fluffy.

Nutrition

Per Serving: 142 calories; protein 1.4g; carbohydrates 9.4g; fat 10.8g; cholesterol 21.1mg; sodium 6.5mg.

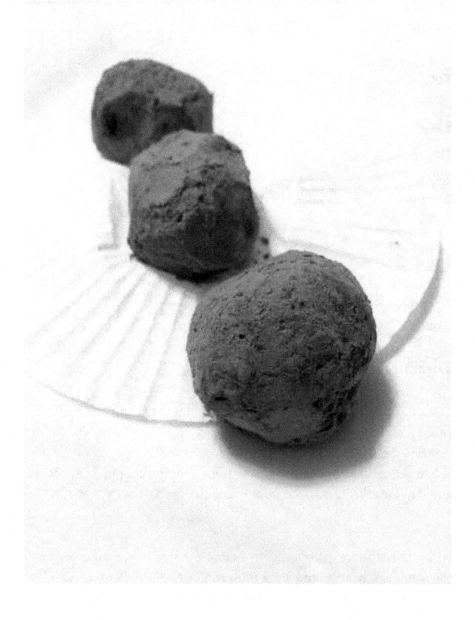

Chocolate Mousse

Prep:

20 mins

Cook:

5 mins

Additional:

4 hrs

Total:

4 hrs 25 mins

Servings:

4

Yield:

4 servings

Ingredients

¾ cup vegan dark chocolate chips
1 tablespoon white sugar
¾ cup aquafaba (chickpea water)

Directions

1

Melt chocolate in top of a double boiler over simmering water, about 5 minutes. Remove from heat and let cool.

2

Beat aquafaba in a stand mixer on high speed until firm peaks form, 10 to 15 minutes. Add sugar gradually into the mixture while continuing to beat. Fold in cooled chocolate gently.

3

Spoon mousse into small glass cups and chill in the refrigerator for at least 4 hours before serving.

Nutrition

Per Serving: 250 calories; protein 3.2g; carbohydrates 28.6g; fat 19.1g.

Pumpkin Cookies

Prep:

20 mins

Cook:

20 mins

Additional:

40 mins

Total:

1 hr 20 mins

Servings:

36

Yield:

3 dozen

Ingredients

2 ½ cups all-purpose flour

1 teaspoon baking soda

2 teaspoons ground cinnamon

½ teaspoon ground nutmeg

½ teaspoon ground cloves

1 teaspoon baking powder

½ teaspoon salt

½ cup butter, softened

1 egg

1 teaspoon vanilla extract

2 cups confectioners' sugar

3 tablespoons milk

1 ½ cups white sugar

1 cup canned pumpkin puree

1 teaspoon vanilla extract

1 tablespoon melted butter

Directions

1

Preheat oven to 350 degrees F. Combine flour, baking powder, baking soda, cinnamon, nutmeg, ground cloves, and salt; set aside.

2

In a medium bowl, cream together the 1/2 cup of butter and white sugar. Add pumpkin, egg, and 1 teaspoon vanilla to butter mixture, and beat until creamy. Mix in dry **Ingredients**. Drop on cookie sheet by tablespoonfuls; flatten slightly.

3

Bake for 15 to 20 minutes in the preheated oven. Cool cookies, then drizzle glaze with fork.

4

To Make Glaze: Combine confectioners' sugar, milk, 1 tablespoon melted butter, and 1 teaspoon vanilla. Add milk as needed, to achieve drizzling consistency.

Nutrition

Per Serving: 122 calories; protein 1.2g; carbohydrates 22.4g; fat 3.2g; cholesterol 12.9mg; sodium 120.5mg.

Strawberry Scones

Prep:

20 mins

Cook:

16 mins

Additional:

20 mins

Total:

56 mins

Servings:

8

Yield:

8 servings

Ingredients

1 cup ripe strawberries - cleaned, hulled and diced

½ cup light cream

2 cups all-purpose flour

⅓ cup white sugar

1 tablespoon baking powder

1 teaspoon vanilla extract

1 ½ teaspoons lemon zest

6 tablespoons cold unsalted butter

½ teaspoon salt

¼ teaspoon ground nutmeg

Directions

1

Preheat oven to 425 degrees F. Line a baking sheet with parchment paper.

2

Place diced strawberries on paper towels to absorb liquid. Combine the cream with the vanilla extract in a small pitcher, and set aside.

3

Whisk the flour, sugar, baking powder, salt, nutmeg, and lemon zest together in a mixing bowl. Cut the cold butter into chunks and add to the flour mixture. Use a pastry blender to cut in butter until mixture resembles coarse, pea-sized crumbs. Stir in strawberries, and gently toss **Ingredients**. Make a hole in the middle of the flour mixture; pour cream mixture into the hole. Quickly stir dough together until just blended. Allow dough to rest 2 minutes.

4

Turn dough out onto a lightly floured work surface; and knead until smooth and satiny, 4 to 5 minutes. Transfer dough to prepared baking sheet and pat into an 8-inch round. Use a serrated knife to cut the round into 8 wedge-shaped pieces. Separate wedges on the baking sheet, leaving at least 1/2 inch space between each.

5

Bake in preheated oven until tops are light brown and crusty, 16 to 18 minutes. Transfer to a wire rack, and cool 20 minutes before serving.

Nutrition

Per Serving: 232 calories; protein 3.5g; carbohydrates 34.3g; fat 9g; cholesterol 22.9mg; sodium 390.4mg.

Japanese Cheesecake

Prep:

35 mins

Cook:

45 mins

Total:

1 hr 20 mins

Servings:

8

Yield:

8 servings

Ingredients

1 (3 ounce) package cream cheese

3 tablespoons all-purpose flour

¼ cup milk

2 egg whites

⅓ teaspoon cream of tartar

1 ½ tablespoons cornstarch

2 egg yolks

¼ cup white sugar, divided

Directions

1

Preheat the oven to 350 degrees F. Line the bottom of a 9 inch round cake pan cake pan with parchment paper.

2

Warm the cream cheese and milk in a small saucepan over medium-low heat. Cook, stirring occasionally, until cream cheese is melted. Remove from the heat and set aside.

3

In a medium bowl, beat egg yolks and half of the sugar until light and fluffy using an electric mixer. Fold the cream cheese mixture into the yolks. Sift in the flour and cornstarch, and stir until blended.

4

In a separate bowl, using clean beaters, whip egg whites with cream of tartar until they can hold a soft peak. Gradually sprinkle in the remaining sugar and continue whipping to stiff peaks. Fold egg whites into the cream cheese mixture. Pour into the prepared cake pan. Place the pan on a baking sheet with sides.

5

Place the baking sheet with the cheesecake into the oven, and pour water into the baking sheet until it is half way full. Bake for 21 minutes in the preheated oven, then reduce the heat to 300 degrees F. Continue to bake for 15 more minutes. Let the cake cool before removing from the pan.

6

Run a knife around the outer edge of the cake pan, and invert onto a plate to remove the cake. Peel off the parchment paper and invert onto a serving plate so the top of the cake is on top again.

Nutrition

Per Serving: 99 calories; protein 2.9g; carbohydrates 10.8g; fat 5g; cholesterol 63.5mg; sodium 50.7mg.

Italian Panna Cotta

Prep:

5 mins

Cook:

10 mins

Additional:

4 hrs

Total:

4 hrs 15 mins

Servings:

6

Yield:

6 servings

Ingredients

⅓ cup skim milk

½ cup white sugar

2 ½ cups heavy cream

1 ½ teaspoons vanilla extract

1 (.25 ounce) envelope unflavored gelatin

Directions

1

Pour milk into a small bowl, and stir in the gelatin powder. Set aside.

2

In a saucepan, stir together the heavy cream and sugar, and set over medium heat. Bring to a full boil, watching carefully, as the cream will quickly rise to the top of the pan. Pour the gelatin and milk into the cream, stirring until completely dissolved. Cook for one minute, stirring constantly. Remove from heat, stir in the vanilla and pour into six individual ramekin dishes.

3

Cool the ramekins uncovered at room temperature. When cool, cover with plastic wrap, and refrigerate for at least 4 hours, but preferably overnight before serving.

Nutrition

Per Serving: 418 calories; protein 3.5g; carbohydrates 20.2g; fat 36.7g; cholesterol 136.1mg; sodium 45.8mg.

Posset

Prep:

5 mins

Cook:

10 mins

Additional:

5 hrs

Total:

5 hrs 15 mins

Servings:

5

Yield:

5 servings

Ingredients

3 cups heavy cream

3 lemons, juiced

3 tablespoons additional heavy cream for topping

1 ¼ cups white sugar

Directions

1

In a saucepan, stir together 3 cups of cream and sugar. Bring to a boil, and cook for 2 to 4 minutes. Stir in the lemon juice. Pour into serving glasses, and refrigerate until set, about 5 hours. Pour a little more cream over the tops just before serving.

Nutrition

Per Serving: 730 calories; protein 3.9g; carbohydrates 61.2g; fat 56.3g; cholesterol 207.9mg; sodium 59.6mg.

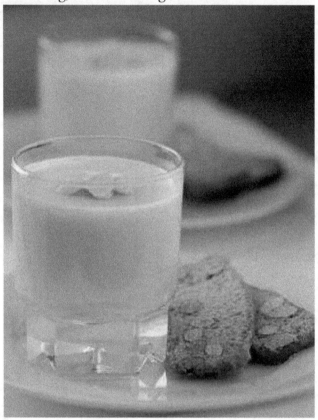

Snickerdoodle Cookies

Prep:

15 mins

Cook:

12 mins

Additional:

3 mins

Total:

30 mins

Servings:

24

Yield:

24 cookies

Ingredients

1 ⅓ cups gluten-free all-purpose flour

1 ½ teaspoons ground cinnamon

1 teaspoon baking powder

¼ teaspoon salt

½ cup butter at room temperature

1 cup sugar, divided

1 egg

¼ teaspoon baking soda

Directions

1

Preheat the oven to 350 degrees F. Line 2 baking sheets with parchment paper.

2

Combine flour, baking powder, salt, and baking soda in a bowl.

3

Whisk butter and 3/4 cup sugar with an electric mixer in a separate bowl until soft and creamy, about 2 minutes. Add egg; whisk until well combined. Add flour mixture gradually; whisk on low speed until a soft dough is formed, about 2 minutes. Shape dough into 1 1/2-inch balls.

4

Combine remaining 1/4 cup sugar with cinnamon in a bowl. Roll balls in cinnamon mixture and place on the prepared baking sheets.

5

Bake in the preheated oven until edges are golden, 12 to 15 minutes. Cool on the baking sheet for 1 minute before removing to a wire rack to cool completely.

Nutrition

Per Serving: 95 calories; protein 1.1g; carbohydrates 14.1g; fat 4.3g; cholesterol 17.9mg; sodium 87.8mg.

Heavenly Keto Caramels

Prep:

15 mins

Cook:

15 mins

Total:

30 mins

Servings:

48

Yield:

48 bars

Ingredients

16 graham crackers

¾ cup brown sugar

¾ cup butter

1 teaspoon vanilla extract

2 cups sliced almonds

2 cups miniature marshmallows

2 cups flaked coconut

Directions

1

Preheat oven to 350 degrees F. Line a 10x15 inch jellyroll pan with aluminum foil.

2

Arrange graham crackers to cover the bottom of the prepared pan. In a small saucepan, combine the butter and brown sugar. Cook over medium heat, stirring occasionally until smooth. remove from the heat and stir in the vanilla. Sprinkle the marshmallows over the graham cracker crust. Pour the butter mixture evenly over the graham crackers and marshmallows. Sprinkle the coconut and almonds evenly over the marshmallows.

3

Bake for 14 minutes in the preheated oven, until coconut and almonds are toasted. Allow the bars to cool completely before cutting into triangles. Store at room temperature in an airtight container.

Nutrition

Per Serving: 114 calories; protein 1.5g; carbohydrates 10.4g; fat 7.9g; cholesterol 7.6mg; sodium 52.8mg.

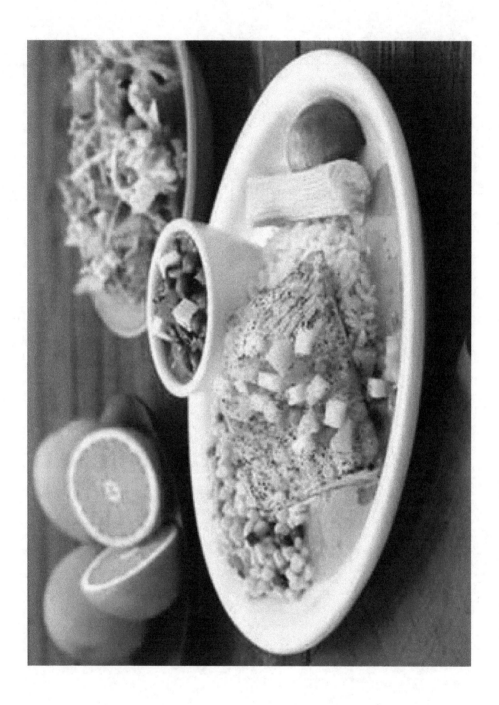

CPSIA information can be obtained
at www.ICGtesting.com
Printed in the USA
BVHW091020300421
605944BV00027B/735